MW01169418

The Little Book of Horse Poop

A collection of tips, truths and tributes

by Becki Bell

Palfrey Media Publishing
Rough and Ready, CA

Contents

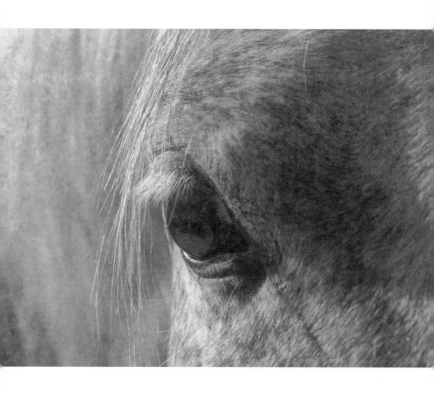

INTRODUCTION

Our horses reward us in so many ways. They greet us with soft noses and nickers, they carry us down overgrown trails, past speeding cars, and over streams, they help us win ribbons and their beauty brings tears to our eyes. In return, we have one simple, yet monumental task to perform: mucking out.

It is one of the great inevitabilities of horse ownership. Every day, we set our teeth and head out to the barn, rake in hand. No matter how you look at it, mucking out will never be the best part of horse ownership. But does it have to be the worst part? Isn't it time we celebrated manure in all its fascinating incarnations?

Manure has been a mainstay of civilization for as long as horses have enjoyed the comforts and trials of domestication. Manure has left its mark on the history books, it has inspired the world's great thinkers, it helps us grow our roses, and it lives on as one of the most maligned and misunderstood substances in our world.

If you didn't already appreciate the many nuances of your horse's manure, this book will help you see that every wheelbarrow of horse poop has its own special place in the world. And that alone, I hope, will help to make your daily chore a little more tolerable. If only just a little.

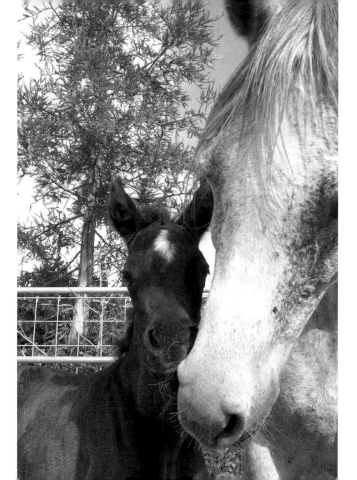

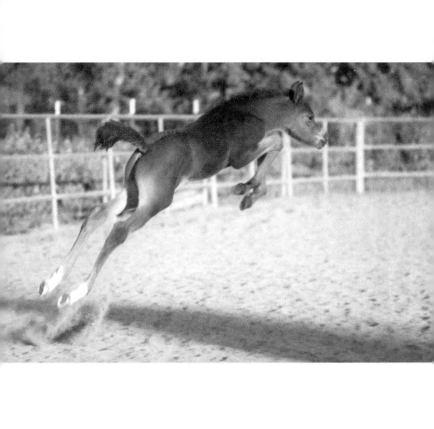

1. HORSE POOP IS INTERESTING

Twelve bits of horse poop trivia
(Some useful, some not)

1

The Poop on Manure

It may surprise you to hear that the word manure does not stem from a root word meaning "excrement." In fact, the word "manure" comes from the Middle English "manuren," meaning "to cultivate land." "Manuren," in turn, stems from the French "main-oeuvre," which means "hand work." This suggests that, in days of old, manure was far too useful to be considered solely on the basis of where it came from.

2

Horses are Poop Machines

On average, a single 1,000 pound horse generates 50 pounds of manure each day (taking an average of three weeks to produce its own weight in poop). That's 18,000 pounds per year, and 450,000 pounds over an average horse's 25-year lifespan.

Poop is Only Slightly Thicker than Water

Horse manure is only 25% solid. The other 75% is water.

4

Raking up the Cash

If all the horse manure produced by all the horses in the United States was properly composted as fertilizer, it would have an annual dollar value of $147.3 million. This means that America's horses are producing potential fertilizer at a dollar value rate of $15 per second.

5

Exploding Poop

Horse manure generates so much heat as it decomposes that large piles of it have been known to spontaneously combust.

6

Oh, Deer

For some reason, deer dislike horse manure. Though they will quite happily eat vegetables, herbs and other garden plants that have been fertilized with chicken and cow dung, they turn their noses up at plants fertilized with horse manure. Savvy gardeners learned long ago to use horse manure not only as a fertilizer, but also to keep deer away from their cherished plants.

7

What Goes in Must Come Out

The horse is a very inefficient food process-
ing machine. Only 4/5ths of what the
horse eats is actually utilized; the rest is
passed out in the horse's manure. This is why
horse manure makes such a good fertilizer.
When manure-based fertilizer is applied to a
field, about half of the nutrients will be used
in the first growing season. The remainder of
those nutrients will stay in the soil and will
be used in subsequent seasons.

8

Papermaking

Horse manure makes a surprisingly good base for paper. If you think you might like to take up this hobby, follow these instructions for your own unique brand of farm stationery:

Soak dried manure overnight. Place the manure in an old pillowcase and hose it down. Then cook the manure in soda ash for two hours. Rinse well and pulverize in a kitchen blender. The end-product can now be used in a paper mold just like any other paper pulp.

9

Wedding Decor

The carriage horses employed for the wedding of Prince Charles and Lady Diana were fed pastel colored dyes so their manure would match the wedding's color scheme and therefore look more aesthetically pleasing on television.

10

Alternative Fuel

When horse manure burns it generates more than half as much heat as charcoal, and slightly more heat than wood.

11

The San Francisco Street

In San Francisco, it is still illegal to pile horse manure more than six feet high on any street corner.

12

Cheap Sports Gear

Hockey has been Canada's national sport for many years. In the early days, the country's abundance of horses meant an abundance of hockey pucks for Canadian children. During the winter months, horse manure would freeze solid, thus becoming inexpensive and effective hockey pucks.

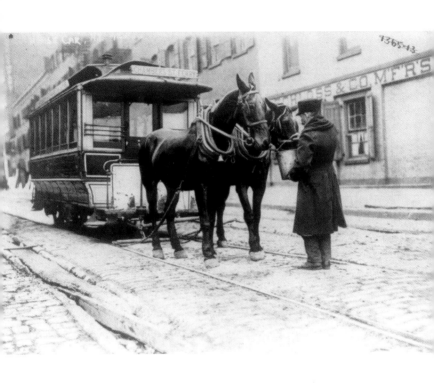

2. HORSE POOP IS A HISTORICAL TREASURE

16 contributions to world history

1

A Pioneer of Flight

In 1783, two French inventors successfully launched the world's first practical balloon. Made from paper and cloth, the balloon was fueled by a combination of chopped wool, straw and horse manure. As the mixture burned, it released hot air, which caused the balloon to inflate and rise. The balloon stayed aloft for eight minutes and landed safely two miles from the launch site. Everyone on board (a sheep, a duck and a rooster) survived.

2

The Great Horse Manure
Crisis of 1894

In the late 1800s, most big cities still depended on horses for transportation and commerce. New York alone had a population of 100,000 horses, which produced 2.5 million pounds of horse manure each day. In London, horse manure was such a problem that in 1894 one writer estimated it would take a mere 50 years before every street in London would be buried beneath nine feet of horse poop.

3

An Alchemist's Recipe

Ancient alchemists may not have known how to turn base metals into gold, but they did know a few things about horse poop:

> "If you would make a heat with horse dung ... make a hole in the ground. Then lay one course of horse dung a foot thick, then a course of unslaked lime a foot thick, and then another of dung, as before. Then set in your vessel, and lay around it lime and horse dung mixed together. Press it down very hard ... When it ceases to be hot, then take it out and put in more."
>
> – "The Art of Distillation" by John French, 1651.

4

Crossing Sweepers

There was so much manure in big city streets that enterprising children would offer up their services as "crossing sweepers," meaning that wealthy pedestrians would pay them to walk several paces ahead with a broom to clear a path through the manure.

5

Roman Poop Looters

Chariot racing was one of the great national pastimes in ancient Rome. Fans of the races would go to great lengths to learn any small piece of information that might help determine the outcome of a race. One favorite tactic was looting the manure. The manure left by chariot racers could tell a bettor which horses were healthy, well-fed, and therefore more likely to win a race. This was such a valuable predictor that many historians believe Rome actually had a thriving black market in horse poop.

6

The Frugal Jockey's Low-Cost Sauna

Manure generates heat as it decomposes, so much heat, in fact, that depression era jockeys used fermenting piles of horse manure as pseudo-saunas. Jockeys eager to "make weight" would don rubber suits, dig holes in the manure pile at their local track, and bury themselves inside in order to burn off extra pounds before a race.

7

A Thing of Beauty

The Santa Clara and San Ildefonso pueblos of New Mexico are famous for producing beautiful black pottery. In order to achieve the black finish, the fire is smothered using a technique that has been passed down through generations. To create an oxygen-free environment, the artists cover the outside of the kiln with tin or metal, then they add a thick layer of horse manure. The manure keeps out the oxygen, ensuring that each piece has a beautiful black finish.

8

Home Sweet Horse Poop

In simpler times, horse manure was one of the world's most abundant resources. It could be used as a wood substitute during lean winters, when fuel for the fire was scarce. Mixed with clay and straw, it also made an inexpensive building block. The manure mixture was poured into molds and allowed to harden, after which it could be used for the construction of surprisingly sturdy houses.

9

Ovens are so Overrated

In The Modern Cook, published in 1735, chefs were advised to:

> "Take a good ham, cleanse it from all the nastiness about it, take off the rine, spread a cloth, in one end of which you put thyme, sweet basil, and bay leaves: then put upon it the ham, the fat side downwards, season it top and bottom alike, adding cloves and pepper. Lay one fold of the cloth over it, besprinkle it with some glasses of brandy, fold it up... Then bury it in horse dung during forty hours, the dung being two foot diameter all round, and two foot deep top and bottom. After that time, you take it out, and serve it up like another ham."

10

Cellar Insulation

The London & Country Brewer, published in 1736, recommended using horse manure to keep cellars temperate for the storage of ale or malt liquor. "... in Winter time, when the Weather is frosty, shut up all the Lights or Windows into such Cellars, and cover them close with fresh Horse-Dung, or Horse-Litter."

11

Ancient Poop

Scientists are using traces of ancient horse manure to revise earlier timelines for horse domestication. A Copper Age site in northern Kazakhstan contains the remains of structures thought to be ancient horse corrals, and the phosphorus-enriched soil inside those corrals indicates that horses may have left their droppings there up to 5,600 years ago.

12

Poopslide

Just one decade after it was built, the old Tijuana racetrack's manure pile was so enormous that it dwarfed even the track's largest structures. The problem of what to do with all that poop solved itself in the late 1920s, when a freak rainstorm picked up the whole pile and used it to wipe out the nearby railroad tracks and the grandstands.

13

The World's First Airborne Missiles

Ancient warfare was, if nothing else, at least innovative. Enterprising weapons designers put petroleum, liquid pitch and oil of sulphur in a pottery jar and buried it in horse manure for fifteen days. They then smeared the resulting substance on crows and flew them into the enemy camp by night. When the sun rose the next morning, the crows would catch fire, thus spreading the flames throughout the enemy's tents.

14

Bellcasting

Bellcasting foundries in England still use many of the same techniques passed down through generations. Among these is the practice of making a mixture (loam) out of clay and horse manure, which is used to create the mould shapes into which the molten metal is poured.

15

When Fuel is Scarce

Early settlers in Saskatchewan, Canada, sometimes made "coal" out of horse manure:

"Horse manure and straw were spread on level ground in a circle of about 30 ft. circumference. This was wetted down with water. With two horses and three harrows, we walked round and round until this was packed solid like brick. This was left about a week or ten days, to bake in the hot sun ... then piled like a pyramid or igloo to shed water so the rain would not soak it ... We used a couple of bricks in a small heater and they burned all night."

– Emmanuel Felske, settler

16

Manure Banking

Older and poorly built houses in the turn-of-the-century midwest often had to be "banked" in the wintertime. This meant piling manure up against the outside walls to help insulate the residents against the cold. The thickness of the manure was usually in direct proportion to the disrepair of the house.

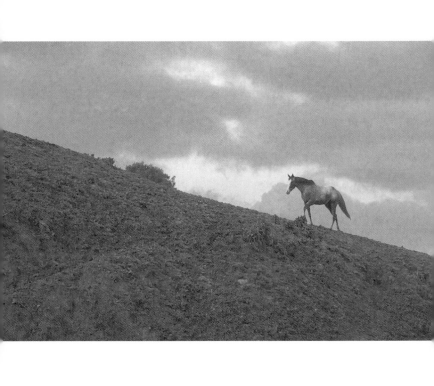

3. HORSE POOP IS LITERARY

Twelve thoughts from great thinkers

1

The Inventor

Nature does have manure and she does have roots as well as blossoms, and you can't hate the manure and blame the roots for not being blossoms.

– Buckminster Fuller

2

The Poet

Humanity is the rich effluvium, it is the waste and the manure and the soil, and from it grows the tree of the arts.

– Ezra Pound

3

The Novelist

The longer I live the greater is my respect
for manure in all its forms.

– Elizabeth von Arnim

4

The Philosopher

If only we were good plowland we would allow nothing to go unused, and in every thing, event, and person we would welcome manure, rain, or sunshine.

– Friedrich Nietzsche

5

The Politician

I do not waste my time in answering abuse; I thrive under it like a field that benefits from manure.

– Henry Labouchere

6

The Cowboy

Sometimes you have to step in it to learn how to avoid it.

– Anonymous

7

The Texas Financier

Money is like manure. If you spread it around, it does a lot of good, but if you pile it up in one place, it stinks like hell.

– Clint W. Murchison

8

The Editor

The civilization of one epoch becomes the manure of the next.

– Cyril Connolly

9

The Merchant

Making money selling manure is better than losing money selling musk.

– Egyptian Proverb

10

The Jazz Singer

They think they can make fuel from horse manure. Now, I don't know if your car will be able to get 30 miles to the gallon, but it's sure gonna put a stop to siphoning.

– Billie Holiday

11

The Folk Artist

In Ukraine we call [manure] Ukrainian gold
because when you spread it on the land it
produces the wheat we turn into bread.

– Sergei Shapoval

12

The Country Western Star

You got to have smelt a lot of mule manure before you can sing like a hillbilly.

– Hank Williams

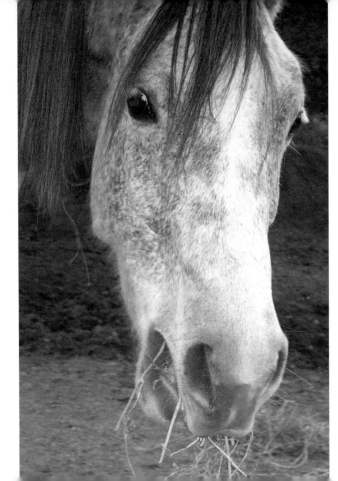

4. HORSE POOP IS VALUABLE

Four weird ways horse poop
became someone's cash cow

1

Olympic Roses

Olympic gold medal winning gelding Shear L'Eau earned £760.00 (about $1,392 US) for charity when the BBC auctioned off his manure on eBay. The auction received a total of 37 bids (starting at £.50), and the lucky winner received some truly gold-medal quality fertilizer.

2

Real Kentucky Manure

A Louisville, KY gift shop sells bags of "Genuine Kentucky Thoroughbred Horse Manure" for $3.75 a bag, billed as a "Party Kit" for a Kentucky Derby Party. Visit www.derbygifts.com for the scoop on this poop.

3

"Turd Birds"

California artist and entrepreneur K. Engelmann sells decorative "Turd Birds" on her website, www.turdbirds.com. The birds' bodies are made from "genuine California horse excrement," dried and sealed in liquid plastic. The legs and necks are made from wood. Note: Engelmann also sells "Poo Ponies."

4

Poo Vacs

The innovative UK based company Trafalgar Cleaning Equipment sells a product called the "Paddock Cleaner," which is essentially a gas-powered vacuum with a large storage container and a 5-inch pick-up hose – just the right size for horse poop. Now, instead of using a shovel or manure fork to pick up all that poop, you can simply vacuum it up. For information about this product, visit www.paddockcleaner.co.uk.

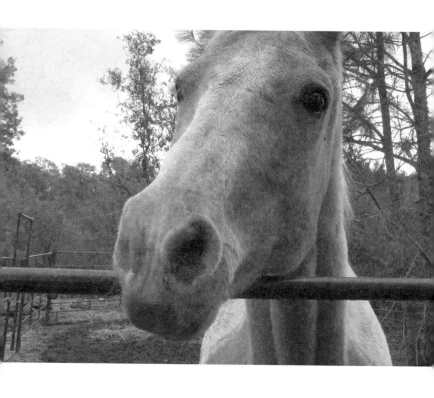

5. HORSE POOP IS NOT EVIL

Four common misconceptions
about horse poop

1

Horse Poop Spreads Disease

On the contrary, horse manure is far cleaner than dog, cat or human poop. You cannot catch West Nile, cryptosporidium, giardia, salmonella or any other insidious disease from handling horse manure.

2

Horse Poop Spreads Weeds

Most horses aren't fed weeds, and even horses that spend a lot of time at pasture don't tend to consume a lot of weeds, since pastures are usually planted with more palatable plants. Even if your horse does eat weeds, seeds of any kind spend too much time in a horse's gut to be good for much upon exit. If you need an example of this process at work, feed your horse whole oats. When you look in his manure, you'll see what appears to be undigested oats, but closer inspection will reveal only empty hulls.

3

Horse Poop on Public Trails can Contaminate Groundwater

Unlike cow and pig excrement, horse poop dries relatively quickly. Once deposited, an isolated pile of horse manure will decompose very quickly, disappearing completely in approximately 12 days. The ammonia and nitrogen content of the manure is lost long before it has a chance to seep into the ground water.

4

Horse Poop on Public Trails
will Encourage the Growth of Weeds

Because the nitrogen in horse manure volatizes so quickly, the random piles of horse manure likely to be found on public trails simply do not contribute enough nutrients to the soil to create favorable growing conditions for weeds.

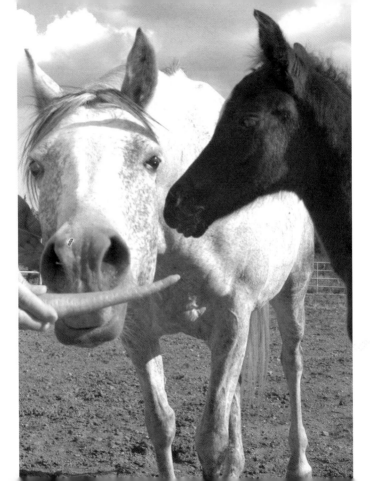

6. HORSE POOP IS FUN

10 ways to make mucking out more
interesting (or at least a lot less sucky)

1

Muck with a Book

No, you don't need to carry a novel in one hand and your manure fork in the other. Instead, buy some books on CD or rent books on tape from the local library. Just as a good story can make a rainy afternoon fly by, a good book might actually make you look forward to your least favorite part of horse ownership.

2

Muck with a Friend

If you have horse-owning neighbors or friends, try sharing mucking-out duties. Your friend can come to your place twice a week to help you clean up after your horses, and you can think of excuses why you can't make it to her house twice a week. Or, if you want the arrangement to last, you could try spending an equivalent amount of time help-ing build her manure pile. Don't forget to gos-sip. Mucking out with a friend is only half as much fun if you behave yourself.

3

Talk your Spouse or Kids
into Helping you

Put on your best concerned parent/spouse face and sit your family down for a heart-to-heart. Tell them you think more together time would be good for everyone. Then tell them mucking out is a great way for you to spend quality time with each other. See if they think you're serious.

4

Offer a Half-Lease as Payment for Mucking-out Duties

If you have an extra horse or you can't ride every day, consider trading a half-lease for mucking out duties. You'd be amazed at how many horseless horse lovers would gladly pick up poop with their bare hands if it meant a chance to ride. Beware, though, and educate yourself about liability laws first. Have a liability release written by a qualified lawyer, and use common sense about who you lease any horse to, especially your half-insane stallion or Bucky-McBuck, the crotchety gelding you haven't dared put a saddle on in four years.

5

Put a Rock in your Shoe

The discomfort of the rock will help you get your mind off of the discomfort of moving poop around.

6

Think of it as Quality Time with your Horses

Scratch their butts with the manure fork. Pet them. Have long one-sided conversations about what you did yesterday and what you had for breakfast, and watch them flick their tails and roll their eyes as they suffer the torment of having to listen to you. Just like your kids.

7

Think of it as Therapy

Horse poop is a great listener, and it doesn't charge $150 an hour. Furthermore, scooping and dumping is a perfect metaphor for ridding yourself of your worries and complaints.

8

Turn up the Radio and Sing

Your neighbors will think you're crazy, and so will your horses. On the up side, a talent scout from a popular record label may drive by. On the down side, he will probably keep on driving by. Last time I checked, mucking-out and pop music were not particularly compatible art forms.

9

Play "Road Apple Barrel Ball"

With your manure fork, lift one road apple. Have your friend, spouse, or offspring push a wheelbarrow around the paddock as fast as he/she can manage (make sure the resident horse is either completely bomb-proof or absent). Chase after the wheelbarrow and attempt to flick the poop inside. Note: while this game can be great fun, it will take a very long time to clean your paddock this way, and by that time the horse en-residence will have filled it with poop many more times over. Fun, but not very efficient.

Advertise it as a way for Frazzled Parents to get their Eight-Year-Old Daughters to Stop Asking for a Pony

Nothing will shatter a little girl's dream of cantering down the beach with the wind in her hair faster than six or seven wheelbarrows full of horse poop. Some parents may actually pay you for this. Another caution, though: horse crazy kids seldom have horse sense—if you have children help you clean paddocks, be sure the horses are not in the paddocks at the time. Someone might get kicked.

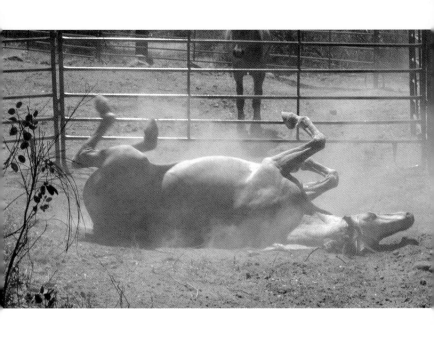

7. HORSE POOP IS USEFUL

Seven ways to make manure management
more manageable

1

Break it Up

If your horses are pastured, you can remove tempting breeding grounds for flies and parasites by breaking up or harrowing the manure with a tractor. This will help the manure dry faster, which in turn will keep any grass unfortunate enough to be right underneath a pile from succumbing to ammonia poisoning.

2

Compost it

Horse manure is valuable because it is rich in nitrogen and ferments easily. With a little effort, you can turn your pile into profit:

Choose a high, level site. Build the pile up to at least three feet. Turn regularly, or insert five-foot PVC pipes (drill holes a few inches apart along the length of each pipe) to help air flow. Cover with a tarp. Keep damp but not soggy. In one to three months the finished compost will be evenly textured and crumbly. Correctly done, composting can reduce the size of your pile by 40 to 60 percent.

3

Use it in your Arena

Perhaps you've spent a lot of time and effort trying to keep manure out of your arena. It may then surprise you to hear that it might be a good idea to put it back, once it's been properly composted. In fact, composted manure can actually improve the footing in your sand arena.

4

Sell it

Organic farmers, gardeners and landscape professionals may actually buy your compost. Compost has value as fertilizer and as a high-quality soil amendment. It is also a useful soil conditioner, improving the drainage of soil as well as its ability to hold nutrients.

5

Spread it

In case you don't have the time or the stomach for composting, you can use a manure spreader to bypass the composting process and add broken up manure directly to your pasture. Your soil will receive fertilizer and you won't have the headache of having to tend to your compost pile. The drawback to manure spreading is that you may reintroduce parasites into your grazing areas, so your horses will need to be on a regular deworming program if you are going to do this.

6

Unload it on Someone Else

Give your manure away to hobby farmers and gardeners. If you are lucky, you may even be able to sell it. Most of the time, you'll be able to get takers to come haul the stuff away, too.

7

Use it for Landscaping

If your property suffers from highs and lows, you can use your manure for land leveling. Simply find the low spots and deposit your manure there. Once the low spot becomes level, cover it with a thin layer of topsoil.

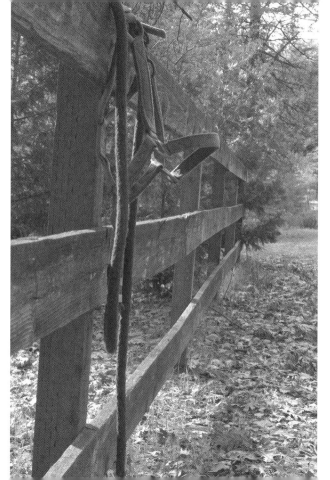

Index

Acknowledgements

Every reasonable effort has been made to acknowledge the creators and copyright holders of images and other material appearing in this book. Any errors or omissions that have inadvertently occurred will be corrected in subsequent editions, provided that the publisher is notified in advance.

All images appearing in this book are copyright B. Bell, except for the following:

22   Bain News Service, N.Y.C., 1908

Do you have a mucking-out tip, or do you know some fun manure trivia? Send email to horsepoop@palfreymedia.com. Your suggestion might appear in the next edition of this book.

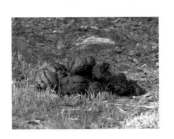